LOSE THE WEIGHT:

Mistakes people make when trying to lose weight and how to avoid them

Carlos k. lewis

Lose the weight

Table of content

Chapter 1: Lose the weight

It's no secret that America has a weight problem. According to the CDC, nearly three-quarters of us are overweight or obese. Yet more than 160 million Americans are on a diet at any given time, and we drop more than $70 billion each year on commercial weight-loss plans, supplements, and other pound-shedding measures. That suggests that losing weight is not easy—yet it is entirely possible when done right.

There are two keys to success when it comes to weight loss. The first is to find an approach that works for you specifically, one that makes you feel good and keeps you motivated. The second is to take your time—sustainable weight loss happens slowly but steadily.

Before you set out on your effort, make sure you know exactly what you're trying to achieve. Ask yourself, "How much weight do I need to lose to be healthy?" Then set personalised goals, in achievable increments and introduce lifestyle changes to gradually lose weight and keep it off.

Be prepared to adapt your lifestyle as necessary to maximise your chances of success.

Weight loss is challenging, especially when you feel like you are doing everything right but not seeing results.

By now, most people are aware that you need to consume fewer calories and exercise more to lose weight. But if you aren't seeing any positive changes, it could be that you are following misguided advice.

5 mistakes to avoid when trying to lose weight.

1. Eating late-night food

One of the most important reasons to avoid late-night eating is the possible risk of weight gain associated with this habit.

While most people are aware of the fact that late-night gorging may contribute to weight gain, they are not always aware of how it can happen. This is caused by the changes in the rate at which our metabolism functions during our sleeping hours versus our waking hours.

At night, our metabolism slows down and the food that we consume is metabolised and digested at a much slower rate.

This may contribute to increased weight, and thus obesity. So people trying to lose weight should eat at least 2 hours before bed. If you must eat late due to unavoidable reasons, then choose foods that are low in calories and rich in fibre.

2. Not eating a balanced diet

To lose weight effectively, your diet needs to be sustainable. Getting enough protein is extremely important if you're trying to lose weight. Protein has been shown to help with weight loss in several ways. It helps boost satiety and build muscle mass, which will help you lose body fat.

It can reduce appetite, increase feelings of fullness, decrease calorie intake, increase metabolic rate, and protect muscle mass during weight loss.

 Also, processed low-fat or "diet" foods are often considered good choices for losing weight, but they may have the opposite effect.

Many of these products are loaded with sugar to improve their taste.

For instance, one cup (245 grams) of low-fat, fruit-flavoured yoghourt can contain a whopping 47 grams of sugar (nearly 12 teaspoons).

Rather than keep you full, low-fat products are likely to make you hungrier, so you end up eating even more.

Instead of low-fat or "diet" foods, choose a combination of nutritious, minimally processed foods.

3. Eating too often, even if you're not hungry

For many years, the conventional advice has been to eat every few hours to prevent hunger and a drop in metabolism. Unfortunately, this can lead to too many calories being consumed over the day. You may also never truly feel full.

In one study, blood sugar levels and hunger decreased while metabolic rate and feelings of fullness increased in men who consumed 3 meals versus 14 meals within a 36-hour time frame.

The recommendation to eat breakfast every morning, regardless of appetite, also appears to be misguided. One study found when people skipped breakfast; they took in more calories at lunch than when they'd eaten a morning meal. However, they consumed an average of 408 fewer calories for the day overall.

Eating only when you're hungry seems to be the key to successful weight loss.

However, letting yourself get too hungry is also a bad idea. It is better to eat a snack than become ravenously hungry, which can cause you to make poor food decisions.

4. Not staying hydrated

Water makes up over two-thirds of a healthy body and plays a significant role in determining your body mass and overall weight.

I advise people who want to lose weight to always drink warm water every morning on an empty stomach because cleanses your bowels, flushes toxins from the body, helps to renew your body, and helps in reducing weight. etc

Dehydration affects how your body burns fat, encourages excessive calorie intake, and slows down your metabolism. It also causes a drop in your energy level, leading to increased tiredness that makes it difficult to be active.

5. Following a Liquid Diet:

Those who wish to lose weight with minimal effort often opt for a liquid diet. This is another weight loss mistake people make.

Replacing healthy meals with green juices, fruit juices, and smoothies will not provide your body with all the essential nutrients. Juices lack fiber and protein, which are key nutrients in keeping you full.

Moreover, fast-food smoothies and prepackaged juices are often loaded with artificial sugar, preservatives, and harmful chemicals.

Drinking prepackaged juice will raise your blood sugar level, leading to hunger and overeating.

Chapter 2:

What metabolism is and how it affects your weight loss

You no doubt have heard of metabolism and may even have a vague idea of what it is. But there are a lot of myths related to the impact metabolism has on your health, especially in terms of weight loss.

In simple terms, metabolism is the internal process by which your body expends energy and burns calories. It runs 24/7 to keep your body moving, even when you're resting or sleeping, by converting the food and nutrients you consume into the energy your body needs to breathe, circulate blood, grow and repair cells, and everything else it does to survive.

This process works at different intensities in different people. How fast your metabolism works is determined mostly by your genes.

"People might have fast, slow, or average metabolism, regardless of their body size and composition," says Dr. Chih-Hao Lee, professor of genetics and complex diseases at Harvard's T.H. Chan School of Public Health.

Age also affects metabolism, as it can slow over the years, even if you start with a fast metabolism. Differences in metabolism speed are evident in how easy or hard it is for people to gain or lose weight. A slow metabolism burns fewer calories, which means more gets stored as fat in the body; that is why some people have difficulty losing weight by just cutting calories. A fast metabolism burns calories at a quicker rate, which explains why some people can eat a lot and not gain extra pounds.

But you can't entirely blame a sluggish metabolism for weight gain, says Dr. Lee. "The reality is that metabolism often plays a minor role," he says. "The greatest factors as you age are often poor diet and inactivity."

Is it possible to speed up a naturally slow metabolism, or rev up one that has become sluggish over time? "You can manipulate your metabolism to a degree," says Dr. Lee. "It is often a small change that may help you burn more calories.

That, along with adopting a healthier diet and making sure you get enough exercise, may give people the extra push they need to lose and maintain weight." For example:

Pick up the pace. Add some high-intensity interval training to your routine. After a period of interval training, your metabolism can stay revved up for as much as a full day. For example, when you're walking or jogging on a treadmill or outside, speed up for 30 to 60 seconds, and then slow to your usual pace; repeat the cycle for eight to 12 minutes.

Eat protein and do weight training. Your metabolism increases whenever you eat, digest, and store food, a process called the thermic effect of food. Protein has a higher thermic effect compared with fats and carbohydrates because it takes longer for your body to burn protein and absorb it.

It's not clear how much of an effect protein has on metabolism, but studies suggest the best approach is to combine adequate protein intake with weight training, which increases muscle mass — and that also can boost metabolism. Use this online calculator to determine your exact daily amount of protein.

Drink green tea. Studies have found green tea contains a compound called epigallocatechin gallate, which may increase the calories and fat you burn. A 2011 meta-analysis published in *Obesity Reviews* found that consuming about 250 milligrams of epigallocatechin gallate (the amount in about three cups of green tea) helped boost metabolism enough to burn an average of 100 extra calories a day.

Get a quality night's sleep; lack of sleep is one of the causes of obesity. It also increases sugar levels and insulin resistance and this increases your risk of developing type 2 diabetes.

Don't joke with your night's sleep.

NOTE: When it comes to weight, metabolism *is* important and does have a genetic component. Whether you can change your metabolic rate, however, is a matter of considerable debate. You *can* change how you balance the calories you take in against the calories you burn up through activity, which can change your weight.

Chapter 3: healthy foods you should focus on as you work on losing weight.

Eat these foods to lose weight and to improve your health in general.

1. Fruits

Beyond being a great option for smoothies or a snack, fruits are jam-packed with many different vitamins and antioxidants.

Opt for fruits like apples, blueberries, bananas, oranges, strawberries and pineapple.

"Fruit can be high in natural sugar and carbohydrates, but portion control is the key. A serving of fruit is about 4 ounces or just under 1 cup of fruit. Fruit can satisfy that sweet tooth without any added sugar or cravings.

2. Vegetables

Turn to veggies like spinach, broccoli, Brussels sprouts, peas, and cauliflower, which are full of fiber.

That fibre expands in your stomach making you feel full so you can cut back on your main course portions to accommodate the extra calories.

"Keep in mind that vegetables are the lowest calorie food group, providing an average of 25 calories per serving, while the majority of the carbs in fruit are in the form of fibre, which isn't digested or absorbed therefore it's eliminated in the form of waste. Vegetables are considered a free food, meaning you can eat unlimited amounts and still lose weight."

3. Whole grains

Oats, brown rice, quinoa — these are just some examples of how you can add whole grains to your meals. A source of fiber and protein, whole grains are a good choice when planning your meals.

Research shows that eating whole grains can help with weight loss.

Don't confuse whole grains with refined grains like white bread, rice pasta, and baked goods. Those are OK to eat in moderation, but they don't provide the same nutritional value as whole grains.

"The fibre and protein in whole grains help you feel fuller, can stabilise blood sugars, and can be very satisfying, which all can lead to meeting your weight loss goals.

4. Legumes

Whether they're dried, canned, or frozen, eating beans and lentils is a smart move.

Options like chickpeas, black beans, lentils, and kidney beans are great replacements for red meat or poultry if you're looking for a meatless meal. Research shows that eating more meatless meals can support weight loss.

"Legumes are a great way to get in protein when you are opting for a lighter meal. Add beans to a salad, stir-fry, burrito, or pasta dish instead of meat for a dose of protein, B vitamins, and potassium.

5. Plant-based oils

There are a lot of options out there when it comes to plant-based oils like olive, avocado, sunflower, grape seed, or peanut.

By using these oils, you'll get the benefit of monounsaturated fat, a healthy fat. Research shows that extra virgin olive oil can improve your cardiovascular health.

If you're baking, sautéing, and grilling, consider peanut oil or avocado oil.

Plant-based oils contain more mono- and polyunsaturated fatty acids, which have been shown to decrease cholesterol, blood pressure, weight, and inflammation when used to replace saturated or animal fats like butter, lard, cheese, sour cream, mayonnaise, and cream.

6. Avocados

Avocado toast is popular for a reason.

This unique fruit boasts a healthy amount of monounsaturated fat, fibre, and water. So, not only does eating it help you feel fuller for longer, but research shows that avocado also helps our body absorb important vitamins like vitamins A, D, E, and K.

"Avocado can be used to replace unhealthy fats like cheese on a salad, mayonnaise, or even butter on toast.

7. Lean protein

Don't overlook lean sources of protein like seafood, skinless poultry, eggs or egg whites, and tofu.

Not only do these options help you feel satisfied, but they can also help you build and maintain muscle. The USDA recommends that 10% to 30% of your calories each day come from protein.

An easy calculation for your personal protein needs is half of your body weight in grams of protein. For example, if you weigh 150 pounds, your minimum protein need is around 75 grams, give or take some depending on your activity and eating preferences.

"Protein is the macronutrient responsible for muscle and tissue rebuilding and repair. If you're exercising, it's very important to eat enough protein to rebuild muscle that is broken down during exercise, especially resistance exercises.

8. Nuts and seeds

Add nuts like pistachios, walnuts, pecans, and almonds to salads, or eat a handful as a snack.

In addition to being a great option to help keep your heart healthy, they contain protein, fiber, and healthy fats. Research indicates that eating nuts can help promote weight loss.

"Nuts can be a great snack. They're filling, crunchy and portable. Keep nut intake down to one ounce per day for weight loss. The calories can add up quickly.

9. Calcium-rich foods

Milk does the body good, right? The calcium found in milk not only helps build strong bones and teeth, but according to research, calcium can also help with weight loss.

Calcium may boost metabolism by increasing your body's core temperature.

So, in addition to milk consider eating other calcium-rich foods like low-fat yoghourt and cottage cheese.

Consider dairy alternatives for calcium if dairy isn't for you. Try fortified tofu, or a dairy-free milk alternative such as almond, soy, coconut, or oat milk or yogurt. Leafy greens, broccoli, almonds, and the bones of salmon also contain calcium.

Eating habits that may promote overweight:

1. Eating few or no meals at home

.

2. Opting for high-fat, calorie-dense foods

3. Opting for high-fat snack foods from strategically placed vending machines or snack shops combined with allowing insufficient time to prepare affordable, healthier alternatives.

4. Consuming meals at sit-down restaurants that feature excessive portion sizes or "all-you-can-eat" buffets

Simple changes that can modify the eating environment :

Lose the weight

1. Prepare meals at home and carry bag lunches

2.   Learn to estimate or measure portion sizes in restaurants

3. Learn to recognize the fat content of menu items and dishes on buffet tables

4. Eliminate smoking and reduce alcohol consumption

5. Substitute low-calorie for high-calorie foods

6. Modify the route to work to avoid a favourite food shop

7 health benefits of drinking warm water on an empty stomach in the morning.

- Cleanses your bowels; drinking water on an empty stomach helps in cleansing the bowels.
- Flushes toxins from the body
- Prevents headaches

Lose the weight

- Helps to renew your body
- Prevents and cures disease
- Helps in reducing weight
- Rehydrate your body.

Chapter 4: Benefits of walking for weight loss

Walking is an excellent kind of exercise for beginners. Since it is free, easy, and available to everyone, walking is the ideal kind of physical activity. You don't need anything fancy or a certain degree of fitness and you can do it just about anywhere. The advantages are vast, ranging from better physical health to enhanced emotional well-being. There is no required degree of fitness for walking.

Regular walking offers many potential health benefits, including weight loss. There are a few ways a person can increase the amount of fat they burn while walking, including wearing a weighted vest and walking uphill.

The American College of Sports Medicine recommends that individuals get at least 150 minutes per week of moderate physical activity. This equates to a total of five sessions each week, consisting of thirty minutes each. The Centers for Disease Control and Prevention (CDC) suggests that individuals obtain at least 150 minutes of this type of activity per week to boost cardiovascular health and lessen the risk of other chronic diseases.

Lose the weight

It's recommended to begin with three shorter walks of ten minutes each and gradually increase the length of your walks until you reach thirty minutes once you feel comfortable doing so.

When you embark on walking, you unveil a treasure trove of wonder that you may never have imagined. As simple as walking is, which is often dismissed by many as not a serious enough exercise, each step tells a story - a captivating one - that reveals hidden rewards and concealed advantages. Come with me, and let us walk the pages of this book together and discover the benefits of walking that extend far beyond what you may have initially thought.

Also adding extra weight to a workout will burn more calories.

A person with more weight will burn more calories because their body requires more energy to perform the same task than someone with less weight; wearing a weighted vest while walking encourages a person's body to work harder during a walk.

One study concluded that individuals, who walked at 2.5 miles per hour (mph) on a flat surface while wearing a weighted vest that weighed 15% of their weight, burned 12% more calories than those who did not wear a vest.

A person wearing a weighted vest that represented 10% of their body weight and who walked at the same pace on a 5-10% gradient burned an average of 13% more calories.

Another study suggested that weighted vests do not change a person's gait negatively. Sometimes it may improve a person's gait.

Though a weighted vest may help burn extra calories, a person should avoid wearing ankle or wrist weights or carrying weights in their hands. Both practices can lead to muscle imbalance and injury.

Word of encouragement

Make time for it. Just get it done. Nobody ever got strong or got in shape by thinking about it. They did it.

Lose the weight